The Complete Thyroid Cookbook

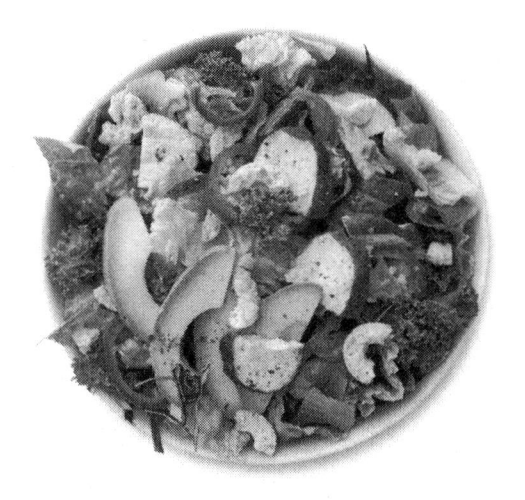

Nourishing Recipes for Hypothyroidism and Hashimoto's Relief

PATRICIA JEFFERS, RDN

Copyright © 2023 by PATRICIA JEFFERS, RDN

All rights reserved. This book or parts thereof may not be reproduced in any form, stored in any retrieval system, or transmitted in any form by any means—electronic, mechanical, photocopy, recording, or otherwise—without prior written permission of the publisher, except as provided by United States of America copyright law and fair use.

Table of Contents

INTRODUCTION 6
THYROID DIET RECIPES 7
BREAKFAST RECIPES 7
   1. Mini Mushroom and Sausage Quiches 7
   2. Coconut Smoothie Bowl 9
   3. Strawberry Rhubarb Baked Oats 11
   4. Beef Taco Bowl 14
   5. Loaded Baked Potato Skins 16
   6. Creamy Mashed Potatoes 18
   7. Sun-Dried Tomato Pesto 20
   8. One-Pot Chicken and Potatoes 22
   9. Slow-Cooked Greens with Garlic 25
   10. Twice Baked Spinach Potatoes 27
LUNCH AND DINNER RECIPES 30
   11. Salmon in Creamy Red Pepper Sauce and Wild Rice . 30
   12. Green Beans with Brown Butter and Pepitas 33
   13. Italian Chickpea Pasta with Sautéed Veggies 35
   14. Almond Crusted Cod with Tropical Salsa 38
   15. Beef Stroganoff 41
   16. Summer Fritatta 45
   17. Shrimp and Potato Chowder 48
   18. Chicken Alfredo Spaghetti Squash Boats 50
   19. Homemade Meatballs with Marinara 53

20. Cheesy Ranch Potatoes 56

21. Skillet-Roasted Chicken with Lemon 59

22. Chicken Fried Steak 62

23. Moroccan Chicken Stew 65

24. Creamy Shrimp Vegetable Skillet 68

25. AIP Cauliflower Fried Rice w/ Basil Khao Pad Kaprow 71

26. Korean Glass Noodle 74

27. AIP Bierocks 78

28. Chicken Kelaguen 83

29. Shepherd's Pie 86

30. Vegan Sauteed Rainbow Chard with Sweet Potatoes and Mushrooms 90

31. Moroccan Chicken 92

32. Southwestern Steak and Peppers 94

33. Sausage, Cherry Tomato and Broccoli Skillet 97

34. Roasted Butternut Squash with Goat Cheese and Pecans 99

35. The Perfect Grain-Free Pizza 101

36. Lemon-Thyme Roasted Chicken Thighs 104

37. Salisbury Steak 106

38. Potato Salad 109

39. Chicken Bacon Pasta Salad 111

40. Dutchess Potatoes 114

SOUP RECIPES 116

41. Cream of Mushroom Soup 116

42. Butternut Squash, Carrot and Coconut Soup 118

43. Tortilla Soup 120

44. Spicy Black Bean Soup 123

45. Indian Chickpea Lentil Soup 126

46. Chicken Pot Pie Soup 128

47. Lemon Chicken and Vegetable Soup 131

48. Butternut Squash Soup 133

49. White Bean Soup with Ham 135

50. Beef Stew 137

INTRODUCTION

Following a diet that is good for your thyroid health can feel restrictive at times and may get to be a little monotonous as you fall into a routine.

Fortunately, it's easy enough to get out of a boring rut. Tons of delicious thyroid-friendly recipes will nourish your thyroid and the rest of your body while also keeping you happy and satisfied.

At the same time, they still use simple ingredients and are relatively easy to prepare.

The recipes in this cookbook contain no gluten or grains which can sometimes be dietary triggers for people with Hashimoto's disease and other thyroid or autoimmune conditions.

THYROID DIET RECIPES

BREAKFAST RECIPES

1. Mini Mushroom and Sausage Quiches
Total: 1 hr 15 mins

Servings: 12

Ingredients

- 8 ounces sausage, turkey, breakfast, removed from casing and crumbled into small pieces
- 1 teaspoon oil, olive, extra-virgin
- 8 ounces mushrooms, sliced
- 1/4 cup scallions (green onions), sliced
- 1/4 cup cheese, Swiss, shredded
- 1 teaspoon pepper, black ground, freshly ground
- 5 large eggs
- 3 large egg whites
- 1 cup milk, lowfat (1%)

Directions

1. Position rack in center of oven; preheat to 325°F. Coat a nonstick muffin tin generously with cooking spray.
2. Heat a large nonstick skillet over medium-high heat. Add sausage and cook until golden brown, 6 to 8 minutes. Transfer to a bowl to cool. Add oil to the pan. Add mushrooms and cook, stirring often, until golden brown, 5 to 7 minutes. Transfer mushrooms to the bowl with the sausage. Let it cool for 5 minutes. Stir in scallions, cheese, and pepper.
3. Whisk eggs, egg whites, and milk in a medium bowl. Divide the egg mixture evenly among the prepared muffin cups. Sprinkle a heaping tablespoon of the sausage mixture into each cup.
4. Bake until the tops are just beginning to brown, 25 minutes. Let it cool on a wire rack for 5 minutes. Place a rack on top of the pan, flip it over and turn the quiches out onto the rack. Turn upright and let cool completely.

2. Coconut Smoothie Bowl

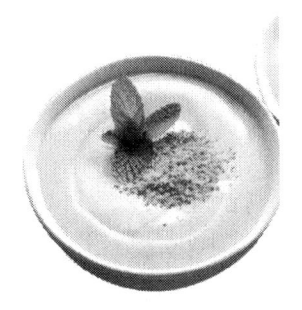

Total: 10 mins

Servings: 1

Ingredients

- 30 g Coconut meat frozen
- 2 tbsp Coconut water
- ½ Banana
- ½ cup Greek yogurt plain non-fat
- 3 Ice cubes or more depending on how cold you want it and the volume you want to add
- ¼ tsp Guar gum optional – to help the smoothie hold toppings

TOPPINGS:

- 1 tbsp Chia seeds
- 1 Kiwi sliced rounds
- 3 Strawberries cut into slices or quarters
- ¼ cup Pineapple diced

Directions

1. Blend all smoothie ingredients, adding only a small amount of coconut water at a time to ensure it is thick enough for toppings to sit on top of and not sink.
2. Pour carefully into a bowl. I used half of a coconut shell as a bowl!
3. Top with the toppings suggested or your own tropical favorites!

3. Strawberry Rhubarb Baked Oats

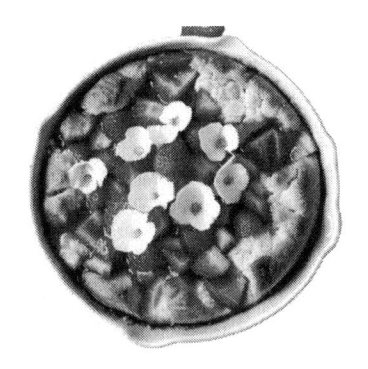

Total: 45 mins

Servings: 6

Ingredients

Dry Mix:

- 2 cup Rolled Oats
- 1 tsp Cinnamon
- 1 tsp Baking Powder
- ½ tsp Salt
- ¼ tsp Nutmeg

Wet Mix:

- 1¼ cup Milk of choice
- 2 tbsp Ground Flax or two eggs minus 1/4 c milk
- 1 cup Applesauce
- 3 tbsp Honey
- 2 tsp Vanilla Extract
- ½ Lemon Zest and Juice

Fruit:

- 2 cup Strawberry
- 1½ cup Rhubarb Pieces

Top:

- ⅔ cup Chopped Pecans
- Greek Yogurt optional, when serving

Directions

1. Cut the strawberries into quarters.
2. Mix all the dry ingredients in a bowl.

3. Mix the milk and ground flax seeds in another bowl, and let it sit for a few minutes.
4. Then add all the other wet ingredients, along with the lemon zest.
5. Pour the wet ingredients into the dry ingredients, and combine them well with a spatula.
6. Grease the cake pan with the oil, and place the strawberries and rhubarb on the bottom.
7. Layer the fruit with the batter.
8. Top it with some pecans.
9. Put it into a preheated oven at 375° F, until it is set and golden brown across the top.
10. Serve it with some fresh strawberries on top and enjoy!

4. Beef Taco Bowl

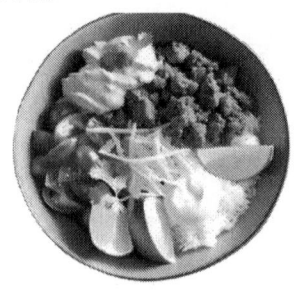

Prep: 10 mins

Cook: 15 mins

Total: 25 mins

Servings: 4

Ingredients

- 2 teaspoons coconut oil or ghee
- 1 yellow onion, diced
- 1 pound ground beef (grass-fed and organic preferred)
- 2 teaspoons ground cumin
- 2 cloves garlic, minced
- 1 teaspoon sea salt

- 3 cups cooked, soaked brown rice or cauliflower rice
- Tomatoes or fermented salsa, avocado, cilantro, sour cream, raw cheese (omit for dairy free), for garnish

Directions

1. Heat coconut oil over medium heat in a large saute pan. Add onion and saute for 5 minutes until soft and just beginning to brown.
2. Add ground beef and cook about 8-10 minutes, breaking up meat with a wooden spoon until no large chunks remain. Make a well in the center of the pan and add the cumin, garlic and salt. Stir spices in the middle of the pan until fragrant, about 30 seconds, and then stir into the meat mixture.
3. Serve meat with rice and toppings of your choice.

5. Loaded Baked Potato Skins

Prep: 25 mins

Cook: 1 hr 20 mins

Total: 1 hr 45 mins

Servings: 4

Ingredients

- 6 large russet potatoes, cleaned
- 2 tablespoons ghee
- 1 tablespoon grey Celtic sea salt
- 4 slices bacon (organic, nitrate-free and pastured preferred), cooked and broken into bits
- 1 1/2 cups raw cheddar cheese, shredded
- 1/2 cup sour cream

Directions

1. Preheat oven to 400 degrees F. Coat each potato with ghee (I use my hands) and sprinkle

generously with salt. Bake in oven for 1 hour or until a knife can be inserted without resistance. Remove from oven and cool for about 10 minutes.

2. Cut each potato in half length-wise and carefully scoop out the flesh (I usually keep this and use for mashed potatoes or potato cakes the next day). Sprinkle each potato skin generously with sea salt. Smear 1 tablespoon of sour cream into each potato skin and top with cheese and bacon.

3. Bake in oven for 10-15 minutes or until cheese is golden and bubbly. Before serving sprinkle with green onion.

6. Creamy Mashed Potatoes

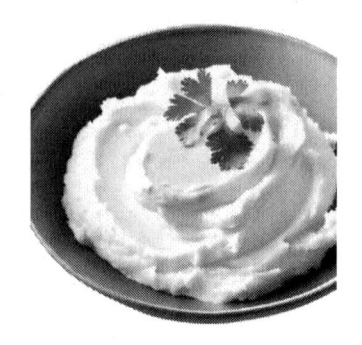

Prep: 15 mins

Cook: 20 mins

Total: 35 mins

Servings: 6

Ingredients

- 3 pounds Yukon potatoes, cut into 2-inch pieces
- 1/2 cup whole milk (I use raw milk)
- 8 tablespoons unsalted butter
- 1/4 cup sour cream

- 1 tablespoon Celtic Sea salt (if you're using a conventional salt like Morton, then add 1 1/2tsp. and then increase the salt to taste)
- Freshly ground black pepper (optional)

Directions

1. Place the potatoes in a large pot, cover with water and bring to a boil over high heat. When the water begins to boil, reduce the heat to medium-high.
2. Continue to boil until potatoes are cooked through, about 15-20 minutes. Drain the potatoes and then put them back into the pot. Add the milk, butter, sour cream and salt to the pot and using a potato masher, mash the potatoes until no large lumps remain.
3. Season to taste with salt and pepper. Serve.

7. Sun-Dried Tomato Pesto

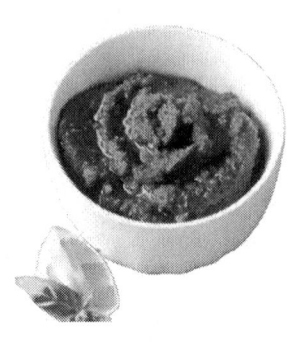

Total: 10 mins

Servings: 1

Ingredients

- 2 cups sun-dried tomatoes in olive oil, drained
- 1 cup soaked and dehydrated walnuts (for a nut-free variation, use toasted sunflower seeds)
- 1 cup Pecorino Romano cheese (omit for a dairy-free option)
- 2 cloves garlic
- 1/2 teaspoon Celtic sea salt
- 3/4 cup extra-virgin olive oil

Directions

1. Place the tomatoes, walnuts, cheese, garlic and salt in the bowl of a food processor.
2. Pulse about 10 times until all ingredients are minced. With the processor on, slowly pour in the olive oil. Adjust salt to taste.

8. One-Pot Chicken and Potatoes

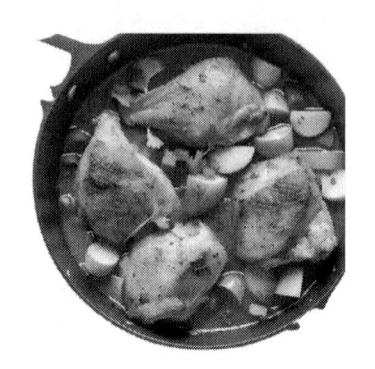

Prep: 10 mins

Cook: 40 mins

Total: 50 mins

Servings: 4

Ingredients

- 3 tablespoons ghee
- Celtic sea salt and freshly ground black pepper
- 8 pieces chicken with skin attached
- 4 russet (baking) potatoes, sliced into 1/4" slices
- 1/4 cup capers, drained
- 5 cloves garlic

- 1 bunch fresh oregano
- 1 teaspoon Celtic sea salt
- 1/2 cup dry white wine (you can substitute with chicken stock)
- 3/4 cup chicken stock
- Juice of 1 lemon

Directions

1. Preheat oven to 400°F and adjust rack to middle position. Heat dutch oven (or a large oven-proof pot) over medium high heat for 2 minutes. Melt ghee in pot and swirl to coat.
2. Season chicken breasts with sea salt and black pepper. Place chicken, skin-side down in the pot and cook until the bottom is golden brown, about 3-5 minutes (the ghee should sizzle when you add the chicken).
3. Using a pair of tongs, remove chicken from the pot and place on a plate (the chicken will not be fully cooked at this point). Place potatoes, capers, garlic, oregano, sea salt, wine and stock in the

dutch oven. Scape any brown bits free from the bottom of the pot (these are full of flavor!).
4. Place chicken on top of potato mixture, put lid on pot and place in the oven. Bake for 10 minutes, remove lid and bake for an additional 20 minutes. Remove from the oven, spritz with lemon juice and serve.

9. Slow-Cooked Greens with Garlic

Total: 35 mins

Servings: 4

Ingredients

- 2 pounds Tuscan kale (you can also use Swiss chard), ribs and stems removed and torn into large bite-size pieces, roughly 2-inches in diameter each
- 4 tablespoons unsalted butter
- 4 cloves garlic, minced
- 1/4 teaspoon red chili flakes
- 1/2 teaspoon Celtic sea salt
- 1 tablespoon fresh lemon juice

Directions

1. Bring a large pot of water to boil. Place the kale in the water and boil for 8 minutes. Drain and then squeeze out the excess water.

2. Melt the butter in a large skillet over medium heat. Add the garlic and red chili flakes and cook until fragrant, about 45 seconds.
3. Add the cooked kale, reduce heat to medium-low and cook, stirring occasionally, for 20-25 minutes until deep green and tender. Remove from the heat and season with salt and stir in lemon juice. Serve.

10. Twice Baked Spinach Potatoes

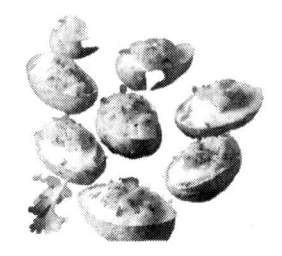

Total: 1 hr 35 mins

Servings: 4

Ingredients

- 4 baking potatoes, cleaned and dried
- 1 tablespoon ghee, melted
- Celtic sea salt for sprinkling
- 1/2 cup butter, softened
- 1/2 teaspoon fresh dill, chopped
- 1/4 cup milk
- 1/4 cup cream
- 1/4 teaspoon freshly cracked pepper
- 1 teaspoon sea salt
- 1 tablespoon sour cream

- 6 cups spinach, cooked down and excess liquid squeezed out (or 1 package of frozen chopped spinach, thawed)
- 1/2 cup parmesan cheese, grated

Directions

1. Preheat oven to 400°F and adjust rack to middle position. Generously oil skins of potatoes with one tablespoon ghee and sprinkle generously with salt. Place the potatoes on a baking sheet lined with unbleached parchment and bake for about 1 hour, until soft.
2. Cut a small slice off the top of potato, scoop out the flesh and place in a large bowl. Arrange empty shells on a baking sheet and place them back in the oven.
3. Add butter, dill, milk, cream, pepper, salt, sour cream, spinach, and 1/4 cup of parmesan cheese in the large bowl with the potato flesh. Mash everything together until combined. Remove the

shells from the oven, turn oven to broil, and then the spoon mixture into crisped shells.
4. Top each potato with remaining 1/4 cup parmesan cheese and broil until cheese is melted and golden brown, about 2-3 minutes.

LUNCH AND DINNER RECIPES

11. Salmon in Creamy Red Pepper Sauce and Wild Rice

Total: 30 mins

Servings: 4

Ingredients

- 4 Salmon filets wild caught
- 2 cups Vegetable broth
- ½ cup Greek yogurt nonfat plain
- ½ cup Milk
- 2 tbsp Arrowroot
- 1 tsp Salt
- ¼ tsp Pepper
- 2 cups Fresh parsley
- ¾ cup Roasted red peppers diced or in strips
- 1/2 Lemon juice, or more if you love lemon
- 3 cloves Garlic
- 1 Onion large

- 1½ tbsp Avocado oil

Directions

1. Heat the pan over medium-high to high with avocado oil.
2. Sear the salmon in a pan 1 minute each side. Remove and set aside.
3. Bring the pan down to low.
4. Add a little more olive oil. Saute the garlic and onion until fragrant.
5. Add broth, milk, seasonings, roasted red pepper and parsley. Bring to a simmer.
6. Add the salmon back to pan and cook until it is done (flip about half way).
7. Stir the arrowroot into yogurt (this prevents the yogurt from coagulating and thickens the sauce).
8. Remove the pan from the heat, and move the salmon to one side of the pan. Stir in the yogurt and arrowroot mixture.
9. Add the lemon juice.

10. To serve: add the wild rice to a plate. Top with the salmon and sauce. Enjoy!

12. Green Beans with Brown Butter and Pepitas

Total: 10 mins

Servings: 4 - 6

Ingredients

- 3 tablespoons unsalted butter
- 1 pound green beans, cleaned and trimmed
- 2 cloves garlic, minced
- 1/2 cup toasted pumpkin seeds (I like to coat them in a little bit of butter and bake at 350 degrees F until golden brown)
- Sea salt and freshly ground black pepper

Directions

1. Melt butter in a large saute pan over medium-low heat until brown and fragrant, about 2-3 minutes, swirling the pan occasionally. Add green beans and toss in the butter until there are spotty brown marks on the beans, about 3-4 minutes.

2. Make a well in the center of the pan and add the garlic. Stir garlic in the center of the pan until fragrant, about 30 seconds and then stir into beans. Remove from heat, toss pumpkin seeds into the beans, then season with salt and pepper to taste. Serve immediately.

13. Italian Chickpea Pasta with Sautéed Veggies

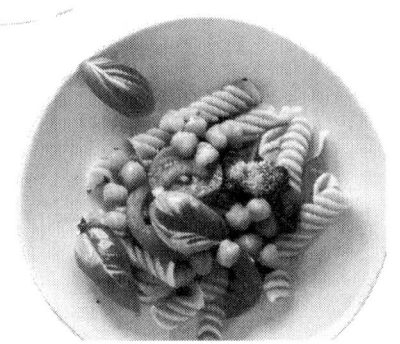

Total: 20 mins

Servings: 4

Ingredients

- 1 box Chickpea pasta
- 1 cup Campari tomatoes quartered or other type
- 1 bunch Asparagus, rough ends removed
- 4 oz Mushrooms, sliced
- ½ Onion, diced
- 1,2 cup Roasted red peppers
- 3 cloves Garlic, minced
- 2 handfuls Fresh basil

- 1 handful Fresh oregano
- ½ cup Olive Oil
- 1 tbsp Butter (or more olive oil)
- ¾ tsp Pepper
- ½ tsp Thyme
- 1 tsp Salt
- 2 tbsp Tahini
- ½ cup Mozzarella or Parmesan cheese or nutritional yeast (for a fully vegan dish) optional, grated

Directions

1. Cook the chickpea pasta.
2. Add some olive oil (or butter) to pan and heat over medium high.
3. Add the asparagus and cover. Rotate occasionally, and cook for about 6 minutes or until the veggies start to soften (not totally cooked!)
4. Remove the cover and add a little bit of the olive oil to the pan.

5. Add the garlic, onion, and mushrooms. Cook until the mushrooms start to soften.
6. Stir in the rest of the olive oil, tahini, fresh basil, fresh oregano, thyme, salt, pepper, roasted red peppers, and tomatoes.
7. Cook for a few more minutes to let the flavors combine together.
8. Serve over the pasta. Enjoy!

14. Almond Crusted Cod with Tropical Salsa

Total: 30 mins

Servings: 4

Ingredients

- 2 lbs Cod wild-caught
- ½ cup Almond Flour

Seasoning Mix:

- ¼ tbsp Garlic powder
- ¼ tbsp Onion powder
- ¼ tbsp Parsley
- ¼ tsp Allspice
- ¼ tsp Black Pepper
- ¼ tsp Cinnamon
- ¼ tsp Cumin
- ¼ tsp Nutmeg
- ¼ tsp Red pepper flakes
- ½ tsp Salt
- ½ tsp Smoked paprika

Tropical Salsa:

- 1 cup Pineapple cubed small
- ½ Mango cubed
- ¼ cup Red onion small dice
- 1 tbsp Lime juice
- 1 Jalapeno minced
- 2 stalks Green onion diced

Directions

1. Prepare the ingredients for the tropical salsa, and add them to a bowl. Set aside.
2. Adjust your oven top rack to be about 4 inches from the heat source. Turn it on high.
3. Mix all the seasonings and the almond flour in a gallon bag.
4. Add the cod a filet at a time and then cover it with the flour seasoning mixture.
5. Spray the grates of a broiling pan with a little bit of oil.

6. Add the fish to the broiling pan and place it on the top rack of the oven.
7. Cook until the fish easily flakes with a fork – it will take about 10-12 minutes.
8. Top the fish with the Tropical salsa.

15. Beef Stroganoff

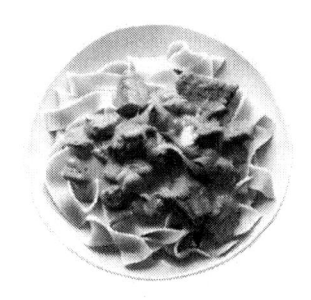

Prep: 10 mins

Cook: 25 mins

Total: 35 mins

Servings: 4

Ingredients

- Celtic Sea salt and freshly ground black pepper
- 1 pound sirloin
- 2 tablespoons ghee
- 12 ounces button mushrooms, cleaned and sliced
- 1 cup chicken broth, divided

- 1 tablespoon unsalted butter
- 1 medium yellow onion, chopped
- 1 teaspoon tomato paste
- 1 teaspoon coconut sugar
- 1 tablespoon arrowroot
- 1/2 white wine (you can sub with chicken broth if needed)
- 1/3 cup sour cream

Directions

1. Generously salt and pepper both sides of the sirloin and then cut into thin strips again the grain, at a sharp 45-degree angle.
2. Heat 1 tablespoon ghee in a large sauté pan over medium heat. Add the mushrooms and cook until the edges are golden brown and they have lost most of their moisture, about 10 minutes. Transfer into a large bowl.
3. Using the same pan, add the remaining ghee. Lay the sirloin pieces in a single layer and brown the sirloin on each side. Be careful not to overcrowd

the pan or they will not brown. Transfer the meat to the bowl with the mushrooms and then repeat with remaining meat.

4. Pour 1/2 cup broth of chicken broth into the now empty pan. Scrape all of the brown bits up from the bottom of the pan and bring the broth to a simmer. Simmer until broth is reduced by half, about 3-4 minutes. Pour the broth into the bowl with the mushrooms and meat.

5. Return the skillet to the stove over medium-low heat. Add the butter. After the foaming subsides, add the onion, tomato paste and sugar.

6. Stir occasionally, and cook for about 6 minutes until the onions turn golden brown. Stir in the arrowroot and continue to stir for about 30 seconds. Add the remaining 1/2 cup broth and the white wine. Bring the sauce to a boil and then reduce to a simmer for 2 minutes.

7. Place the sour cream into a small bowl and add 1/2 cup of the sauce to the sour cream and stir (this step will keep the sauce from curdling). Add the sour cream mixture to the pan, along with the beef and mushrooms. Stir until combined.

8. Season with salt and pepper to taste. Serve over baked potato, or gluten-free egg noodles.

16. Summer Fritatta

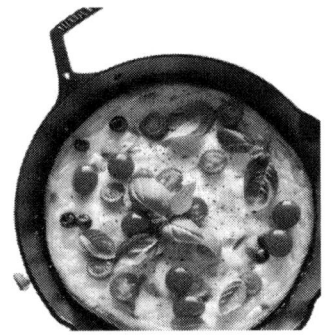

Prep: 15 mins

Cook: 45 mins

Total: 1 hr

Servings: 6

Ingredients

- 1 zucchini, cut into about 1 1/2" pieces
- 1 red, yellow or orange bell pepper, cut into about 1 1/2" pieces
- 1 red onion, cut into about 1 1/2" pieces
- 2 tablespoons ghee, melted
- 4 cups arugula
- 10 eggs

- 1 tablespoon heavy cream
- 1 teaspoon Celtic sea salt
- 1/4 teaspoon freshly ground black pepper
- 1/2 cup grated Pecorino Romano cheese (you can sub with Parmigiana Reggiano)
- 1 cup grated mozzarella cheese

Directions

1. Preheat the oven to 400°F and adjust the rack to the middle position. Place the zucchini, pepper and onion on a large baking sheet lined with parchment paper. Drizzle the ghee over the vegetables and then toss until evenly coated. Spread the vegetables out evenly on the pan. Roast for 20 minutes, until just golden on the edges.
2. Pour the roasted vegetables into a large skillet and top with the arugula. Heat the pan over medium and toss until the arugula is wilted.
3. Whisk together the eggs, cream, sea salt, pepper and Pecorino Romano cheese in a large bowl.

Pour the egg mixture over the vegetables and stir gently to combine. Let the mixture cook for 2 minutes on the stove. Sprinkle the mozzarella cheese overtop and then bake in the oven for 15-20 minutes, or until the chase is just turning golden brown. Cool for 5 minutes and then slice into wedges and serve.

17. Shrimp and Potato Chowder

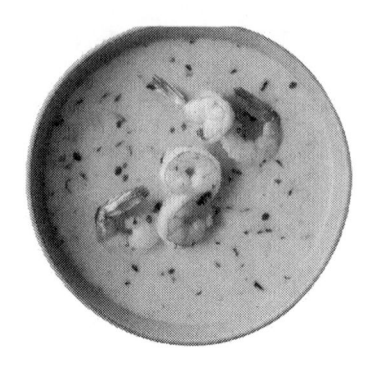

Prep: 10 mins

Cook: 20 mins

Total: 30 mins

Servings: 4 - 6

Ingredients

- 2 tablespoons unsalted butter or coconut oil
- 2 bunches green onions, chopped
- 2 pounds baby potatoes, cut into bite-size pieces
- 6 cups bone broth
- 2 teaspoons Celtic sea salt

- 1 1/2 cups heavy cream (I prefer raw cream, or for a dairy-free option, use coconut milk)
- 1 1/2 pounds wild shrimp
- 4 glugs of hot sauce

Directions

1. Place the butter in a large pot over medium heat. Melt the butter and then add the onions. Cook the onions for 2 minutes, stirring occasionally.
2. Add the potatoes, stock, and salt then bring to a simmer. Cook for about 10-15 minutes until potatoes are fork tender.
3. Stir in the cream and cook until hot (but not boiling). Add the shrimp and cook until no longer pink, about 3-4 minutes. Stir in hot sauce, season to taste and serve.

18. Chicken Alfredo Spaghetti Squash Boats

Total: 1 hr 30 mins

Servings: 4

Ingredients

- 2 spaghetti squash, cut in half length-wise and seeds removed
- 2 tablespoons unsalted butter
- 6 cloves garlic, chopped
- 1/2 teaspoon granulated garlic
- 1 tablespoon arrowroot
- 1 cup whole milk (I recommend raw, but you can also use pasteurized, but non-homogenized)
- 1 cup heavy cream {I recommend raw, but you can also use pasteurized, but non-homogenized)
- 1/4 cup parmesan cheese
- 1 tablespoon Celtic sea salt
- 3 cups cooked and shredded chicken breast
- 1 cup mozzarella cheese, shredded

Directions

1. Preheat the oven to 400°F and adjust the rack to the middle position. Place the 4 squash halves, cut-side down on a baking sheet lined with parchment paper. Bake for 45 minutes. You can do this earlier in the day if needed.
2. Melt the butter over medium heat in a saucepan. Stir in the chopped and granulated garlic, and arrowroot. Whisking constantly, add in the milk and cream, and continue to cook until just starting to thicken, about 5-7 minutes. Whisk in the parmesan and salt. Stir in the shredded chicken.
3. Using a potholder, carefully pick up a spaghetti squash half and, using a fork, scrape the spaghetti squash out of the skin and into a large bowl. Repeat with remaining 3 squash halves. Pour Alfredo sauce over the squash and stir until incorporated. Spoon an even amount of squash mixture back into each of the 4 squash "bowls". Top with mozzarella cheese. Bake for 30 minutes

until mozzarella cheese is turning golden brown and bubbly.

19. Homemade Meatballs with Marinara

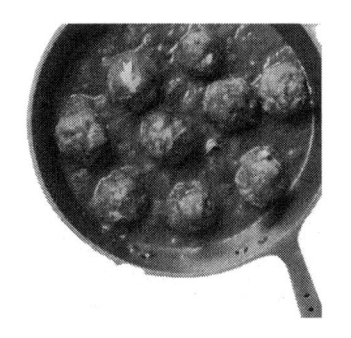

Prep: 15 mins

Cook: 25 mins

Total: 40 mins

Servings: 6

Ingredients

FOR THE MARINARA:

- 2 cloves garlic, minced
- 2 tablespoons extra-virgin olive oil
- 4 large tomatoes, chopped
- 1 teaspoon sea salt

FOR THE MEATBALLS:

- 1 1/2 pounds ground beef
- 2 tablespoons tomato paste
- 1 1/4 cup shredded Pecorino Romano cheese
- 1 teaspoon dried Italian seasoning
- 1 teaspoon sea salt
- 1/4 teaspoon freshly ground black pepper
- 1/4 cup shredded basil leaves

Directions

1. Place garlic and olive oil in a large sauce pan over medium-low heat. Cook until garlic begins to sizzle and is fragrant. Add tomatoes and salt. Simmer the sauce for 10 minutes.
2. Place beef, tomato paste, 1 cup cheese, seasoning, salt and pepper in a large bowl. Using your hands, massage the meat until ingredients are incorporated. Form meat into golf-size balls and place on a large baking sheet. When all of the meatballs have been formed, place the meatballs

into the simmering sauce. Cook for about 10 minutes, until meatballs are cooked through. Top with basil and remaining cheese. Serve immediately.

20. Cheesy Ranch Potatoes

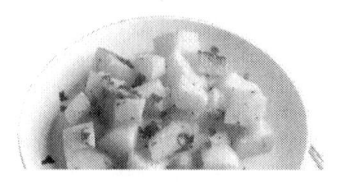

Prep: 15 mins

Cook: 40 mins

Total: 55 mins

Servings: 6

Ingredients

For the potatoes:

- 2 pounds Yukon gold potatoes, cut into 1-inch pieces
- 4 tablespoons ghee or lard, melted
- 1 teaspoon granulated garlic
- 1 teaspoon onion powder
- 1 teaspoon Celtic sea salt
- 1/4 teaspoon freshly ground black pepper

- 2 cups grated cheddar cheese

For the ranch dipping sauce:

- 2 tablespoons whole buttermilk
- 1/4 cup mayonnaise
- 1/4 cup sour cream
- 1/4 teaspoon dried dill
- 1/4 teaspoon dried parsley
- 1/4 teaspoon dried chives
- 1/2 teaspoon garlic powder
- 1/2 teaspoon lemon juice
- 1/8 teaspoon Celtic sea salt

Directions

1. Preheat the oven to 400 degrees F and adjust the rack to the middle position. Place the potatoes in a large 13×9 baking dish and toss with ghee, garlic, onion powder, sea salt and black pepper. Roast the potatoes until they are tender and golden brown on the bottoms, about 30 minutes.

2. Meanwhile, whisk together all of the ingredients for the dipping sauce in a medium bowl. Set aside.
3. Sprinkle the cheese over the potatoes and continue to roast until cheese is melted and bubbly, about 5 minutes. Let it cool for 5 minutes. Drizzle with ranch sauce and serve.

21. Skillet-Roasted Chicken with Lemon

Prep: 15 mins

Cook: 35 mins

Total: 50 mins

Servings: 4 - 6

Ingredients

For the Chicken:

- 3 pounds bone-in chicken pieces (breasts or thighs)
- Celtic sea salt

For the sauce:

- 2 tablespoons ghee, divided (use lard or duck fat for dairy-free)
- 1 shallot, chopped
- 2 garlic cloves, chopped
- 1 teaspoon coconut flour
- 1 cup bone broth or meat stock

- 1/2 teaspoon Celtic sea salt
- 1/4 lemon juice
- Zest from 1 lemons
- 2 tablespoons fresh parsley, chopped
- 1 teaspoon fresh thyme, minced

Directions

1. Preheat oven to 475 degrees F and adjust the rack to the middle position. Sprinkle each chicken thigh with sea salt. Place 1 tablespoon of the ghee in a 12" oven-proof skillet over medium high heat, swirling the pan to coat. Place the chicken skin-side down in the skillet and cook until the skin is browned and crisp, about 8 minutes. Flip the chicken pieces and continue to cook until browned on the second side, about 5 minutes. Transfer chicken to a plate.
2. Reduce the stove temperature to medium and add the remaining 1 tablespoon ghee, shallot and garlic and cook until fragrant, about 45 seconds. Sprinkle the coconut flour over the garlic mixture,

stirring constantly and cook for about 1 minute. Slowly stir in the broth, sea salt and lemon juice, scraping the bottom of the pan to release any browned bits. Bring to a simmer. Stir in the zest and remove from the heat. Place the chicken, skin-side up, in the pan with the garlic mixture and place in the oven. Roast for about 10 minutes until chicken is cooked through.
3. Let chicken rest for 5 minutes, sprinkle with parsley and thyme. Season to taste with sea salt and serve.

22. Chicken Fried Steak

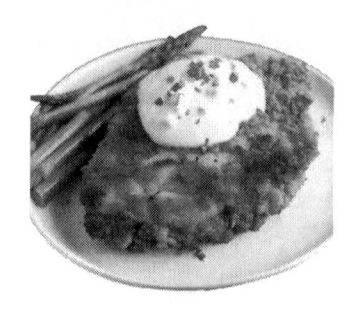

Prep: 15 mins

Cook: 20 mins

Total: 35 mins

Servings: 4

Ingredients

- 2 cups finely ground almond flour
- 1/4 cup coconut flour
- 1 tablespoon Herbamare
- 1 teaspoon paprika
- 1/2 cup arrowroot flour
- 1 1/2 teaspoons grass-fed gelatin
- 5 large eggs

- 4 tenderized cube or round steak
- 1/2 cup lard, tallow or palm shortening

Directions

1. Place a cooling rack on top of a baking sheet. Preheat the oven to 275°F and adjust the rack to the middle position.
2. While the lard is heating, place the almond flour, coconut flour, Herbamare, paprika, arrowroot and gelatin in a pie plate and toss gently to combine.
3. Crack the eggs into a second pie plate and whisk in 2 tablespoons of water. Dip one of the cube steaks first into the flour mixture, then the egg, then the flour again. Set the coated steak on a large plate while you coat the remaining steaks.
4. Place the lard in a large 12" skillet and heat over medium-high heat until the lard is shimmering. Carefully place two steaks into the skillet and fry for about 3-4 minutes until the bottom side is golden brown. Using a pair of tongs, carefully

turn the steaks over to the other side. Fry for another 2-3 minutes until the second side is golden brown. Place the steaks on the prepared baking sheet. Place the sheet into the oven to keep the steaks warm while you cook the remaining steaks. Serve hot.

23. Moroccan Chicken Stew

Prep: 10 mins

Cook: 35 mins

Total: 45 mins

Servings: 8

Ingredients

- 1-2 tbsp olive oil (or oil of choice)
- 2 large sweet potatoes cubed (about 5-6 cups)
- 2 pounds chicken breasts cut into 1" cubes
- 2 cups cauliflower cut into small florets
- 2 cups diced mushrooms
- 2 cups chicken broth
- 1 13.5 oz can coconut cream
- 2 tbsp coconut aminos
- 2 tbsp nutritional yeast
- 1 tbsp turmeric
- 2 tsp garlic powder
- 2 tsp sea salt

- 1/2 tsp ground cinnamon
- 1/4 tsp ground ginger
- 1/8 tsp ground cloves
- fresh cilantro finely sliced (optional garnish)

Directions

1. Heat 1-2 tbsp of oil in a large skillet over medium-high heat. Add the sweet potatoes. Cook for 8-10 minutes.
2. Push the sweet potatoes to one side of the pan and add the chicken cubes to the other side of the pan. Cook for about 8 minutes keeping the chicken and sweet potatoes separate but stirring/flipping them occasionally to keep from sticking/burning.
3. Once the chicken starts to brown a little bit, start to mix the chicken and potatoes together, then add the cauliflower and mushrooms. Cook for another 3-4 minutes.
4. Add in the broth, coconut cream, coconut aminos, and spices. Turn the heat down to medium and

simmer for another 12-15 minutes or until sweet potatoes are tender.
5. Allow it to cool slightly then serve. Garnish with fresh cilantro.

24. Creamy Shrimp Vegetable Skillet

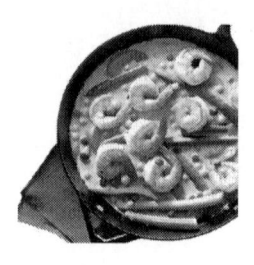

Total: 30 mins

Servings: 2

Ingredients

- 2 tbsp olive oil or avocado oil
- 1/2 cup red onion, diced
- 1 cup asparagus cut into 1" pieces stems discarded
- 1 pound medium-sized shrimp, peeled and deveined
- 3/4 cup +2 tbsp full fat coconut milk, divided
- 1/2 tsp pink sea salt
- 1/2 tsp garlic powder
- 1/2 tsp onion powder
- 1/4 tsp tumeric powder

- 1/4 tsp dried cilantro
- 1/4 tsp dried parsley
- 1/4 tsp coconut sugar omit for Whole30
- 1/2 tsp nutritional yeast
- 1 tbsp arrowroot starch
- 2-3 cups raw spinach

Directions

1. Dry the shrimp with paper towels (Make sure they've been thawed, peeled, and deveined).
2. Heat about 2 tbsp of oil over medium heat in a large pan. Add the onions and saute for 1-2 minutes. Next, add the asparagus and continue cooking and strirring 3-4 minutes until slightly softened (but not too much).
3. Lower the heat to medium. Add the shrimp to the vegetable mixture and cook for 2-3 minutes.
4. Add the coconut milk (reserving 2 tbsp for later) and spices (save the arrowroot starch for later). Stir until everyting is evenly combined.

5. Mix 1-2 tbsp remaining coconut milk with the arrowroot starch, then add to the pan with the other ingredients. Stir in and turn heat to low. Simmer for 3-4 minutes on low to allow the mixture to thicken.
6. Stir in the spinach and allow to wilt; about 2 minutes.
7. Remove from heat and serve.

25. AIP Cauliflower Fried Rice w/ Basil Khao Pad Kaprow

Total: 30 mins

Servings: 4

Ingredients

- 2 tbsp avocado oil or olive oil
- 2-3 cloves garlic minced
- 8 oz boneless skinless chicken breasts, cut into bite-sized cubes
- 2 cups frozen or fresh cauliflower rice
- 1 tbsp fish sauce
- 1 tbsp coconut aminos
- 1/2 tbsp honey or maple syrup (omit for Whole30)
- 1/8 tsp dried ginger (optional)
- 1/8 tsp turmeric (optional)
- pinch (less than 1/16 tsp) ground cloves (optional)
- 2 tbsp shallots
- 1/4 cup fresh basil finely chopped

- 1-2 tbsp fresh cilantro finely chopped

Garnish:

- 2 limes quartered
- fish sauce
- coconut aminos

Directions

1. In a large pan over medium heat, add oil. Heat for 1 minute then add the garlic. Saute the garlic 1-2 minutes until it starts to brown.
2. Add the chicken. Cook for about 5 minutes or until nearly cooked through. Add the cauliflower rice and cook for about 2 minutes or until no longer frozen. If using raw cauliflower, cook until tender.
3. Add the fish sauce, honey, and coconut aminos. Stir until incorporated.
4. Add the shallots, ginger, cloves, turmeric, basil, and cilantro. Cook for about 1 minute then remove from the heat.

5. Serve with lime wedges, coconut aminos, and fish sauce on the side.

26. Korean Glass Noodle

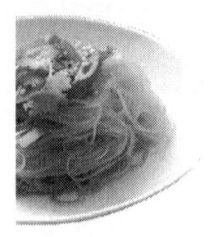

Prep: 15 mins

Cook: 15 mins

Total: 30 mins

Servings: 4

Ingredients

- 1 3.5 oz package of sweet potato glass noodles

Sauce:

- 1/4 cup coconut cream
- 1/2 tsp fresh grated ginger
- 2 tsp lime juice
- 2 tsp white wine vinegar
- 1 tbsp coconut aminos

- 1/4 tsp garlic powder
- 1/4 tsp sea salt
- 1 tsp honey

Main Dish:

- 1 tbsp olive oil
- 1 pound ground beef
- 8 oz shiitaki mushrooms, sliced
- 1/2 tsp onion powder
- 1/2 tsp garlic powder
- 1/2 tsp salt
- 1/2 tbsp white wine vinegar
- 1 tbsp coconut aminos
- 2 carrots, peeled into ribbons
- 1 cucumber, peeled into ribbons

Garnish:

- green onions, thinly sliced
- cilantro, chopped

Directions

1. Mix sauce ingredients until smooth. Set aside.
2. Cook glass noodles according to package instructions. Set aside.
3. In a medium-sized pan over medium to medium-high heat, add oil. Heat for 30 seconds, then add the ground beef. Break up the beef and cook until almost browned (about 5-7 minutes).
4. Add the mushrooms, garlic powder, onion powder, salt, white wine vinegar, and coconut aminos to the pan. Continue cooking an additional 3-5 minutes until mushrooms are softened. Remove from heat.
5. Assemble beef noodle bowls. Start with the noodles, then top with meat/mushrooms, carrots, cucumbers. Drizzle with the sauce and sprinkle with green onions and cilantro.

Tip

- Use a vegetable peeler for carrots and cucumber ribbons

- If noodles cool off after cooking and stick together, add a little bit of water to loosen them up again.
- Leftovers will stay fresh in the fridge for about 3 days- keep the fresh veggies, meat, and sauce separate from each other if possible.

27. AIP Bierocks
Total: 1 hr 5 mins

Servings: 16 rolls

Ingredients

Filling:

- 8 oz ground beef (85% fat or less)
- 1/2 white onion, finely diced
- 3 cups shredded green cabbage
- 1/2 tsp sea salt

Rolls:

- 4 cups yuca root peeled, boiled, and roughly chopped (middle stringy part removed)
- 1 cup coconut flour
- 6 tbsp coconut oil melted
- 1/2 tsp sea salt

Directions

Filling:

1. In a non-stick frying pan over medium-high heat, add the ground beef. Cook for 5-6 minutes or until nearly browned. Drain off any excess grease- this will ensure the bierocks don't get soggy later.
2. Add the onions. Cook for 2-3 minutes or until translucent.
3. Add in the cabbage and salt. Continue cooking the mixture for another ~5 minutes or until the beef is cooked through and the cabbage is tender. Remove from heat and set aside.

Rolls:

1. Preheat the oven to 350 degrees Fahrenheit.
2. In a food processor, add the roll ingredients and blend until smooth. You may notice the mixture starts out a little crumbly however as you keep blending, it will form a cohesive dough. *If you don't have a food processor, you can use a fork or potato masher to start mashing the ingredients

together. You can also use your hands to knead the dough and get it nice and smooth.

3. Take the dough out of the food processor. If you find it's a little too sticky to easily handle, sprinkle a little coconut flour over it as needed until it becomes easy to work with.

4. Place the dough on a piece of parchment paper (if you have it- if not, no worries). Break the dough into 16 even sections and form them into balls. Flatten each piece of dough to about 1/4 of an inch thick and 5 inches in diameter using a rolling pin or your hands. *I personally just used my hands, placed the dough between two sheets of parchment paper and pressed down. This made it a little easier to avoid the dough sticking to my hands. Be careful not to roll them too paper-thin as they will tear.

5. Add about 2 tablespoons of filling to the center of each piece of dough. Then close the dough around the mixture, sealing it inside. You can do this by gathering the edges gradually and pinching the dough together as you work your way around the

piece of dough. It should all pinch together at the top.
6. Once you have the dough gathered at the top, you can pick up the dough ball and cup it in both hands, gently pressing it all together to form a nice round, smooth ball.
7. Place the bierocks on a parchment paper-lined baking sheet and bake at 350 degrees for 35-40 minutes.
8. Allow to cool slightly, then serve. For an additional flavor boost: dip them in a little honey.

Tips:

- The rolls are relatively small (they fit just in the middle of my palm). I'd recommend 3-4 rolls per adult if using as a main meal. This recipe is about the right amount for our family of 4 (2 adults, 2 grade school kids).
- To Freeze: Place in an airtight container for 1-2 months.

- To Reheat from Frozen: Bake in the oven at 350 degrees Fahrenheit for 15-20 minutes (watch closely). OR Heat for 45-60 seconds in the microwave. Internal temp should reach 165 degrees Fahrenheit.

28. Chicken Kelaguen

Prep: 15 mins

Cook: 20 mins

Marinating time: 9 hrs

Total: 9 hrs 35 mins

Servings: 4

Ingredients

- 2 pound boneless skinless, chicken thighs
- Marinade (for raw chicken)
- 1/2 cup coconut aminos
- 3/4 cup white wine vinegar
- 1 cup white or yellow onion, chopped
- Lemon Mixture (for cooked chicken)
- 1/4 cup lemon juice
- 1 bunch green onions, diced (about 6 green onions)
- 1 cup thick coconut flakes, unsweetened

- 1-2 serrano peppers or hot chili peppers, minced (Optional, Omit for AIP)
- 2-3 tbsp full fat coconut milk
- 1/4 tsp sea salt

Directions

1. Mix the marinade ingredients in a medium bowl, add the chicken and make sure it's covered. Refrigerate and allow to marinate for 8 hours or overnight.
2. If you have an air fryer, use the grill setting and preheat the air fryer to low (400 degrees), and set the time to 17 minutes.
3. Once preheated, add the chicken to the air fryer and discard the marinade. Close the lid. Flip it half-way through.
4. (If no air fryer, heat a pan with olive oil over medium-high heat on the stove and cook the chicken for 5-6 minutes per side or until it reaches an internal temp of at least 165 degrees Fahrenheit).

5. Once done cooking, put the chicken on a plate and allow it to cool for about 10 minutes.
6. While the chicken cools, combine the lemon juice, green onions, coconut shreds, coconut milk, and salt.
7. Dice the chicken into small bite-sized pieces and add it to the lemon juice mixture. Stir it well and put it in the fridge to chill for about an hour.
8. Serve with cauliflower rice or Paleo/AIP-friendly pitas/tortillas.

29. Shepherd's Pie

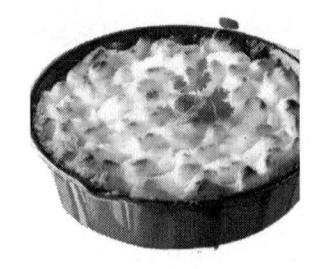

Prep: 20 mins

Cook: 1 hr

Total: 1 hr 20 mins

Servings: 6

Ingredients

Mashed "Potatoes"

- 4 large green plantains
- 3 tbsp coconut oil
- 1 cup water (reserved from boiling the plantains)
- 1 tsp sea salt

Filling:

- 1 tbsp olive or avocado oil
- 1 cup yellow onion, diced (about 1/2 an onion)
- 2 cups carrots, diced small (3-5 medium carrots)
- 2 cups parsnips, diced small (1-2 parsnips)
- 3 cloves garlic, minced
- 1 pound ground beef (less than 15% fat)
- 2 tsp fresh rosemary, finely diced
- 1 tsp fresh thyme, finely diced
- 1 1/2 tsp sea salt
- 1 cup chicken broth or beef broth
- 1/2 tbsp apple cider vinegar
- 1 tbsp coconut aminos
- 1 tbsp arrowroot starch
- 2 tbsp cold water

Directions

1. Bring a medium-sized pot of water to a boil over medium-high heat.

2. While waiting for the water to boil. Peel the plantains. Cut them lengthwise into quarters. Remove the seeds if desired. Cut the quarters in half to form 8 short pieces per plantain. *how you cut the plantains isn't super important- just cut them into small-ish pieces so they boil relatively quickly.
3. Add the plantains to the boiling water. Boil for about 20 minutes or until fork-tender. Set aside when done.
4. Meanwhile, preheat the oven to 400 degrees Fahrenheit.
5. In a medium pan over medium-high heat, heat the oil. Add the onions, carrots, and parsnips. Cook for about 8 minutes or until they start to soften. *Reduce heat to medium if needed.
6. Add the garlic.
7. Add the ground beef and seasonings. Continue stirring occasionally and cook until the beef is browned.
8. Add the broth, coconut aminos, and apple cider vinegar.

9. Make a slurry with the arrowroot starch and water. Add it to the pan with the meat mixture. Cook 2-3 more minutes until the sauce starts to thicken. Remove from heat.
10. Pour the meat mixture into a glass baking dish (8 inch round or 9x11 in). Make sure it's deep enough for the filling and the "potato" topping.
11. Mash the plantains with a fork or potato masher. Add in the water gradually (you may not need the whole cup), along with the coconut oil, and sea salt. Make sure they are nice and thick.
12. Add the mashed plantains to the glass dish on top of the meat mixture. Spread the plantains evenly and all the way to the edges of the dish using a rubber spatula. Form a smooth surface on top.
13. Bake for 20-30 minutes at 400 degrees Fahrenheit or until the plantain surface starts to brown.
14. Remove from the oven and allow to cool slightly. Sprinkle with extra thyme and rosemary for garnish and serve.

30. Vegan Sauteed Rainbow Chard with Sweet Potatoes and Mushrooms

Prep: 10 mins

Cook: 30 mins

Total: 40 mins

Servings: 4

Ingredients

- 2-3 tbsp olive oil or avocado oil, divided
- 2 sweet potatoes diced into 1/4 inch cubes
- 1 bunch rainbow chard chopped, stems and greens separated (about 6-8 large leaves)
- 1 cup raw mushrooms diced
- 1 tsp garlic powder
- 1/2 tsp sea salt
- 1 tsp italian seasoning
- 1-2 avocados diced

Directions

1. Preheat oven to 400 degrees Fahrenheit.
2. Place diced sweet potatoes on a parchment-lined baking sheet. Drizzle with 1-2 tbsp olive or avocado oil and stir until potatoes are evenly coated. Roast for 20-30 minutes checking every 5-10 minutes to stir. Remove from the oven when they are tender and slightly toasted.
3. While sweet potatoes are cooking, dice swiss chard and mushrooms. Be sure to separate the stems of the swiss chard from the greens.
4. Saute the swiss chard stems with 1-2 tbsp olive oil in a medium frying pan over medium-high heat for 3-4 minutes. Add swiss chard greens, mushrooms, and seasonings. Continue to cook for 3-4 more minutes until greens are slightly wilted and mushrooms are tender. Remove from heat.
5. Remove sweet potatoes from the oven and add to the frying pan with the swiss chard and mushrooms. Mix together and serve with diced avocado on top.

31. Moroccan Chicken

Total: 5 hrs 10 mins

Servings: 4

Ingredients

- 2 pounds chicken, pieces (breast halves, thighs, and drumsticks) skinned finely shredded
- 1/2 cup orange juice
- 1 tablespoon oil, olive
- 1 tablespoon ginger, fresh
- 1 teaspoon paprika
- 1 teaspoon cumin, ground
- 1/2 teaspoon coriander, ground
- 1/4 teaspoon pepper, red, crushed
- 1/8 teaspoon salt
- 2 teaspoons orange peel
- 2 tablespoons honey
- 2 teaspoons orange juice

Directions

1. Place chicken in a large resealable plastic bag set in a deep dish. For marinade, in a small bowl, stir together the 1/2 cup orange juice, the olive oil, ginger, paprika, cumin, coriander, crushed red pepper, and salt. Pour marinade over chicken. Seal bag; turn to coat chicken. Marinate in the refrigerator for at least 4 hours or up to 24 hours, turning the bag occasionally.
2. Meanwhile, in a small bowl, stir together orange peel, honey, and the 2 teaspoons orange juice.
3. Drain the chicken, discarding the marinade. Prepare grill for indirect grilling. Test for medium heat above pan. Place chicken, skinned sides up, on lightly greased grill rack over drip pan. Cover and grill for 50 to 60 minutes or until chicken is done (170°F for breast halves; 180°F for thighs and drumsticks); brush occasionally with honey mixture during the last 10 minutes of grilling.

32. Southwestern Steak and Peppers

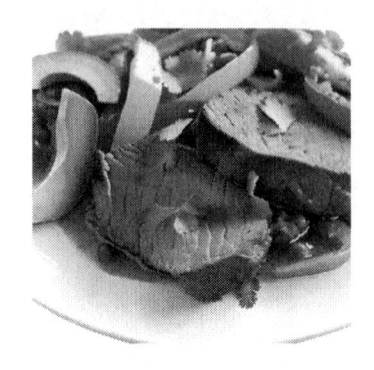

Total: 30 mins

Servings: 4

Ingredients

- 1/2 tablespoon cumin, ground
- 1/2 teaspoon coriander, ground
- 1/2 teaspoon chili powder
- 1/4 teaspoon salt
- 3/4 teaspoon pepper, black, coarsely ground
- 1 pound beef, boneless top sirloin steak trimmed of fat
- 3 cloves garlic, peeled, 1 halved and 2 minced

- 3 teaspoons oil, canola divided (or olive oil)
- 2 medium peppers, red, bell thinly sliced
- 1 medium onion, white halved lengthwise and thinly sliced
- 1 teaspoon sugar, brown
- 1/2 cups coffee, brewed or prepared instant coffee
- 1/4 cup vinegar, balsamic
- 4 cups watercress

Directions

1. Mix cumin, coriander, chili powder, salt, and 3/4 teaspoon pepper in a small bowl. Rub steak with the cut garlic. Rub the spice mix all over the steak.
2. Heat 2 teaspoons oil in a large heavy skillet, preferably cast iron, over medium-high heat. Add the steak and cook to desired doneness, 4 to 6 minutes per side for medium-rare. Transfer to a cutting board and let rest.
3. Add remaining 1 teaspoon oil to the skillet. Add bell peppers and onion; cook, stirring often, until softened, about 4 minutes. Add minced garlic and

brown sugar; cook, stirring often, for 1 minute. Add coffee, vinegar, and any accumulated meat juices; cook for 3 minutes to intensify flavor. Season with pepper.

4. To serve, mound 1 cup watercress on each plate. Top with the sautéed peppers and onion. Slice the steak thinly across the grain and arrange on the vegetables. Pour the sauce from the pan over the steak. Serve immediately.

33. Sausage, Cherry Tomato and Broccoli Skillet

Prep: 5 mins

Cook: 10 mins

Total: 15 mins

Servings:

Ingredients

- 1 tablespoon ghee
- 12 ounces cooked organic Italian sausage, cut into coins
- 2 pints cherry tomatoes
- 2 cloves garlic, chopped
- 1 teaspoon Celtic sea salt
- 1/2 teaspoon dried thyme
- 1/4 teaspoon freshly ground black pepper
- 2 bunches baby broccoli, ends trimmed
- 2 tablespoons unsalted butter

Directions

1. Place the ghee in a large skillet over medium heat and swirl to coat. Add the sausage and cook for 10 minutes, stirring occasionally until lightly browned.
2. Stir in the tomatoes and cook for 5-7 minutes until tomatoes begin to burst (you can also press down on some of the tomatoes with the back of a wooden spoon to encourage the bursting).
3. Add the garlic and cook for about 30 seconds until fragrant. Stir in the salt, thyme and pepper and cook for 1 minute. Add the baby broccoli and then cover with a lid and cook for 3 minutes.
4. Remove from the heat and stir in the butter until melted. Serve immediately.

34. Roasted Butternut Squash with Goat Cheese and Pecans

Prep: 10 mins

Cook: 45 mins

Total: 55 mins

Servings: 6

Ingredients

- 1 2-3 pound butternut squash, skin and seeds removed and cut into 1/2" thick slices
- 3 tablespoons ghee, melted
- 1/2 teaspoon Celtic sea salt
- 1/8 teaspoon cayenne
- 1/4 cup goat cheese, crumbled
- 1/2 cup pecans, toasted and chopped
- 1 teaspoon fresh thyme leaves

Directions

1. Preheat the oven to 425°F and adjust the rack to the lowest position. Place the squash in a large bowl and toss with the ghee, sea salt and cayenne.
2. Spread the squash in an even layer on a baking sheet lined with parchment paper. Roast for 25-30 minutes until well browned. Remove the squash from the oven and, using a pair of tongs, flip each piece of squash. Then, continue to roast in the oven until the face-down side of the squash is browned, about 10 more minutes.
3. Transfer the squash to a platter and top with the goat cheese, pecans and fresh thyme. Serve warm.

35. The Perfect Grain-Free Pizza
Prep: 10 mins

Cook: 30 mins

Total: 40 mins

Servings: 4

Ingredients

- 1 cup water
- 2 cups tapioca flour
- 1/2 cup coconut flour
- 2 teaspoon Celtic sea salt
- 3 tablespoons ghee (or palm shortening for a dairy-free option)
- 2 large eggs (or 2 gelatin eggs for an egg-free option)
- 1 1/4 cups shredded mozzarella cheese (omit for dairy-free)

FOR THE SAUCE:

- 1/2 cup marinara

FOR THE TOPPINGS:

- Pick which ones you prefer such as cheese, pepperoni, bell peppers, olives, onions, etc.

Directions

1. Preheat the oven to 425°F and adjust the rack to the middle position. Line 2 large baking sheets with unbleached parchment paper.
2. Pour the water into a medium saucepan and bring to a simmer. Place the tapioca flour, coconut flour, salt, ghee, eggs and cheese in the bowl of a food processor and pulse to combine. With processor turned on, slowly add the hot water and process until smooth. Let it sit for 5 minutes.
3. Spoon the mixture onto the lined baking sheets, placing 2 mounds on each sheet. Using an offset spatula, spread each mound into an 8-inch round (about 1/4" thick). Bake for 12-15 minutes, or until just golden brown on the edges.
4. Spread 2 heaping tablespoons of marinara on each crust. Top with any toppings you want. Bake

for 10 minutes, or until the cheese is bubbly and just turning golden brown.

36. Lemon-Thyme Roasted Chicken Thighs

Prep: 10 mins

Cook: 20 mins

Total: 30 mins

Servings: 4

Ingredients

- Zest from 1 lemon
- 1 tablespoon fresh lemon juice
- 2 cloves garlic, minced
- 1 tablespoon chopped cilantro
- 1 tablespoon chopped thyme
- 1/2 teaspoon Celtic Sea salt
- 4 bone-in, skin-on organic chicken thighs
- 2 tablespoons ghee , melted (or duck fat for dairy-free)

Directions

1. Preheat the oven to 425°F and adjust the rack to the middle position. Place a wire cooling rack over a baking sheet.
2. Combine the lemon zest, juice, garlic, cilantro, thyme, and sea salt in a small bowl and stir to combine. Loosen the skin on the chicken things and insert about 1 tablespoon of lemon mixture under skin of each.
3. Brush each chicken thigh (bottom and top of thigh) with ghee and place on the wire rack.
4. Roast the chicken until the skin is golden brown and crisp and a thermometer inserted into the thickest part of the chicken, but not touching the bone registers 165°F, about 20-25 minutes. Remove the chicken from the oven and let it rest for 5 minutes. Serve.

37. Salisbury Steak

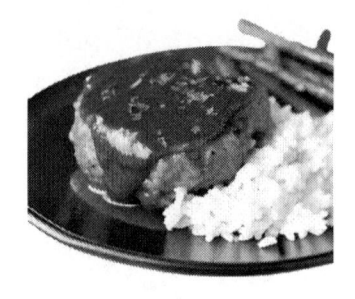

Total: 30 mins

Servings: 4

Ingredients

For the steaks:

- 16 ounces ground beef
- 2 tablespoons chopped green onion
- 1 tablespoon chopped fresh parsley
- 1/2 teaspoon Celtic Sea Salt
- 1/8 teaspoon freshly ground black pepper
- 1 tablespoons coconut flour
- 2 tablespoons arrowroot flour
- 2 tablespoons ghee

For the sauce:

- 1 yellow onion, sliced thin
- 2 cups cremini mushrooms, sliced (you can use white button if desired)
- 2 cloves garlic, minced
- 1/4 teaspoon dried thyme
- 1 tablespoon tomato paste
- 1 cup chicken broth
- 1/2 teaspoon Celtic Sea Salt

Directions

1. Place the beef, onion, parsley, sea salt and pepper in a bowl and use your hands to combine. Divide the beef into 4 oval patties.
2. Place the coconut flour and arrowroot in a pie plate. Dredge each patty in the flour mixture.
3. Heat the ghee in a sauce pan over medium high heat and swirl the pan to coat. Place the steaks in the pan and cook until browned, about 3 minutes

per side. Remove the steaks from the pan and set aside.

4. Place the onions and mushrooms in the now empty pan, reduce to medium, and cook for about 10 minutes, stirring frequently. Stir in the garlic, thyme and tomato paste and cook for 1 minute, stirring frequently. Stir in broth and salt. Place the steaks back in the pan on top of the onion and mushroom mixture.

5. Reduce the heat to medium-low, cover with a lid, and cook for 10 minutes. Adjust salt and pepper to taste. Serve.

38. Potato Salad

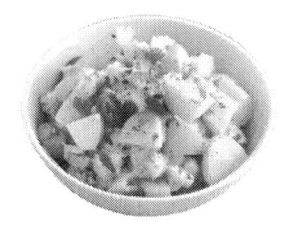

Total: 6 hrs

Servings: 6 - 8

Ingredients

- 3 pounds red potatoes, cleaned, skinned, and cut into 1/2"-thick pieces
- 1 cup fermented pickle juice
- 1/2 cup mayonnaise
- 1/2 cup chopped celery
- 1/2 cup chopped fermented pickles
- 1/2 cup red onion, chopped
- 2 tbs fresh dill, minced

Directions

1. Place the potatoes in a large pot, cover with water, and bring to a simmer over medium-high heat. Cook for about 15 minutes, until tender. Drain.
2. Pour the hot cooked potatoes into an 11×7 baking dish, pour the pickle juice over and gently stir. Cover loosely with plastic wrap and let the potatoes sit at room temperature for about 1 hour to cool.
3. Combine the mayo, celery, pickles, red onion and dill in a small bowl. Pour the mayo mixture over the cooled potatoes and stir to combine. Cover and chill in the fridge for about 4-6 hours. Serve cold.

39. Chicken Bacon Pasta Salad

Prep: 10 mins

Cook: 45 mins

Total: 55 mins

Servings: 6

Ingredients

- 1 pound chicken breasts diced
- 12 oz bacon (precooked weight), cut into small pieces
- 3.5 oz sweet potato glass noodles (1 package= 3.5 oz)
- 1 cup cucumber diced
- 1/2 cup purple cabbage finely sliced
- 1/4 cup red onions minced

Dressing

- 1/2 cup coconut cream
- 2 tsp white wine vinegar
- 2 tbsp lemon juice

- 1/2 tsp dried dill weed
- 1/2 tsp garlic powder
- 1/4 tsp onion powder
- 1/4 tsp salt

Garnish:

- 1/4 cup green onions

Directions

1. Preheat oven to 375 degrees F.
2. Place chicken in a lightly greased glass baking dish and bake for about 35-40 minutes or until internal temeperature reaches 165 degress F
3. While chicken is cooking, fill a small pot with water and place it on the stove over high heat. (this will be for the noodles).
4. While waiting for the water to boil, cook the bacon. Place the bacon in a medium sized pan over medium heat. Continue cooking until bacon is crisp and slightly browned. Scoop the bacon out

of the pan and onto a plate covered with papertowels. Set aside.
5. Once the water for the noodles comes to a boil, cook the noodles according to the package instructions- usually about 5-7 minutes. Once the noodles are cooked, drain the water.
6. Mix the sauce ingredients.
7. Allow chicken to cool before assembling the salad.
8. In a large bowl, combine noodles, chicken, bacon, cucumbers, red onions, and sauce. Stir until well combined and serve.

Tips:

- Allow the chicken to cool before adding it to the salad.
- If the noodles sit for a few minutes, they may stick together a little bit but don't worry- this is easily fixed by adding a little bit of water (a tablespoon or two) and loosening the noodles with a fork.
- This will keep in the fridge for about 3 days in an airtight container.

40. Dutchess Potatoes

Prep: 20 mins

Cook: 40 mins

Total: 1 hr

Servings: 10 - 12

Ingredients

- 4 pounds Yukon Gold potatoes, cut into 2" pieces
- 5 large egg yolks
- 1/2 teaspoon powdered garlic
- 1 cup heavy cream
- 1/2 cup sour cream
- 8 tablespoons unsalted butter
- 1 teaspoon Celtic sea salt

Directions

1. Place the potatoes in a large pot and cover with water. Bring the potatoes to a boil and cook until tender, about 20 minutes. Drain.
2. Preheat the oven to 425°F and adjust the rack to the middle position. Whisk together the yolks, garlic, heavy cream, sour cream, butter and sea salt in a large bowl. Pass the potatoes through a ricer or food mill directly into the egg mixture. Gently stir until combined (don't over mix). Pour the potatoes into a 3-quart baking dish and decoratively shingle or swirl surface. Bake 30-40 minutes until golden brown on top and slightly puffed. Serve.

SOUP RECIPES

41. Cream of Mushroom Soup

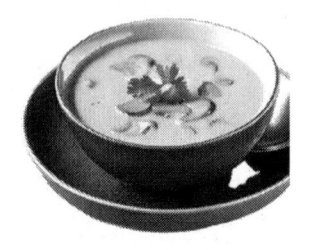

Prep: 5 mins

Cook: 20 mins

Total: 25 mins

Servings: 4

Ingredients

FOR THE SOUP:

- 4 tablespoons unsalted butter

- 1 pound mushrooms, any kind, sliced into 1/4 inch-thick pieces
- 3/4 teaspoon Celtic sea salt
- Few dashes of freshly ground black pepper
- 1 tablespoon arrowroot
- 1 1/2 cups bone broth or meat stock
- 1 1/2 cups heavy cream
- 1 1/2 tablespoons tamari sauce

Directions

1. Melt butter in a medium saucepan over medium heat. Stir in mushrooms, salt and pepper. Cook until mushrooms have released their moisture, about 8 minutes.
2. Add arrowroot while continuously stirring and cook for about 30 seconds.
3. Stir in stock and cream and simmer until soup is thick and reduced, about 10 minutes. Remove from heat, stir in the soy sauce, and serve.

42. Butternut Squash, Carrot and Coconut Soup

Total: 40 mins

Servings: 4 - 6

Ingredients

FOR THE SQUASH:

- 2 pounds butternut squash, peeled, seeded and cut into 2-inch chunks
- 1 tablespoon ghee, melted (you can substitute palm shortening for a dairy-free option)

FOR THE SOUP:

- 2 tablespoons unsalted butter (or coconut oil)
- 3 carrots, cut into 1/4" thick coins
- 1 leek, white and light parts only, chopped
- 1/2 teaspoon dried thyme
- 1 1/2 teaspoons Celtic sea salt
- 3 cups chicken broth (you can use bone broth or meat stock)

- 1 cup coconut milk

Directions

1. Preheat the oven to 400°F and adjust the rack to the middle position. Place the squash on a baking sheet lined with unbleached parchment paper. Pour the ghee overtop and gently toss to coat the squash. Roast for 30 minutes, or until soft when pierced with a knife.
2. Meanwhile, melt the butter in a large pot over low heat. Add the carrots and leeks and stir to combine. Put the lid on the pot and let the vegetables sweat for 30 minutes. After 30 minutes, remove the lid and stir in the thyme and sea salt.
3. Add the chicken broth and roasted squash to the carrot mixture and bring to a simmer. Then, using an immersion blender, blend the soup until smooth. Or, you can also process the soup in a blender until smooth. Stir in the coconut milk. Season to taste with sea salt. Serve.

43. Tortilla Soup

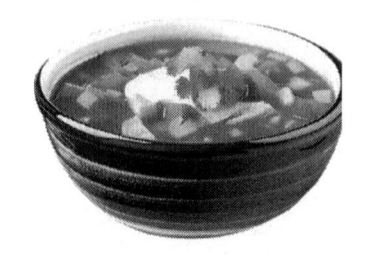

Prep: 15 mins

Cook: 30 mins

Total: 45 mins

Servings: 6

Ingredients

FOR THE SOUP:

- 5 cloves garlic, crushed with skins on
- 6 springs fresh oregano
- 6 sprigs of cilantro, plus 1/2 cup roughly chopped
- 8 cups chicken stock

- 2 pounds bone-in chicken breasts or 1 small 3-4 pound chicken

FOR THE TOPPINGS:

- 3 cups Siete tortilla chips
- 1 avocado, cubed
- 2 tomatoes, cut into bite-size chunks
- 1 lime, cut into quarters
- 1/2 cup sour cream (omit for Paleo and Gaps)
- 1/2 cup shredded cheddar cheese (omit for Paleo)

Directions

1. Place the garlic cloves in a large dutch oven over medium-high heat. Cook, stirring frequently until garlic begins to darken, about 2-2 1/2 minutes.
2. Remove the pot from the heat and let it cool for about 30 seconds and then add the chicken stock, oregano, cilantro, and chicken to the garlic.
3. Place pot back on heat and bring to a boil and then reduce to a simmer. Simmer for about 30 minutes. When chicken is cooked through,

remove the chicken from the broth mixture and set aside.

4. With slotted spoon, strain out the rest of the garlic and herbs. Shred the chicken with a fork and then add back to the soup. Add salt and pepper if needed.
5. To serve, crumble a handful of tortilla chips into individual bowls and then ladle the broth over. Serve with cilantro, avocado, tomatoes, lime, cheese, and sour cream.

44. Spicy Black Bean Soup

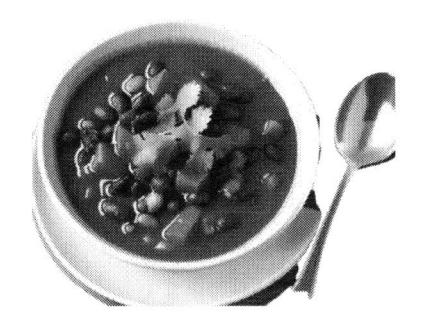

Prep: 10 mins

Cook: 3 hrs

Total: 3 hrs 10 mins

Servings: 6

Ingredients

For the Soup:

- 2 cups black beans, soaked overnight, then drained
- 8 cups beef or chicken stock
- 1 28–ounce can diced tomatoes
- 1 teaspoon paprika

- 1 teaspoon onion powder
- 1 teaspoon garlic
- 1 heaping tablespoon Celtic sea salt
- 1 tablespoon tomato paste
- 1/2 bunch cilantro, plus 2-3 tablespoons more for garnish
- 1 jalapeño pepper, seeded and sliced
- 1 bunch green onions chopped
- Sour cream for serving (omit for dairy free)

Directions

1. Combine beans, stock, tomatoes, paprika, onion powder, garlic, sea salt and tomato paste in a large pot. Bring to a boil, then lower to a simmer and cook for 3 hours.
2. Add cilantro, jalapeño and green onions to soup and let simmer for 5 minutes. Using a hand immersion blender, blend until smooth, or transfer to a blender in batches and blend until smooth.

3. Serve with a dollop of sour cream and sprinkle with cilantro.

45. Indian Chickpea Lentil Soup

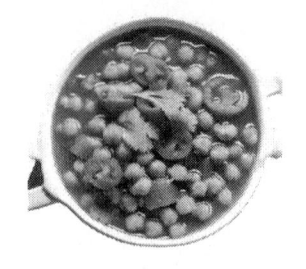

Prep: 10 mins

Cook: 30 mins

Total: 40 mins

Servings: 4

Ingredients

- 1 Onion large
- 3 cloves Garlic minced
- 1 tbsp Olive Oil
- 2 cups Potatoes diced
- 6 cups Vegetable Broth low-sodium
- 1 can Tomatoes diced

- 3 tbsp Ground Flax
- 1 pinch Salt
- ½ tsp Pepper
- 4 Carrots medium-sized, diced
- 1 Red Pepper diced
- ¾ cup Chickpeas dried
- ¾ cup Lentils, green dried
- Indian Blend

Directions

1. Put the olive oil into the instant pot.
2. Add the onion, garlic, carrots, and peppers into the instant pot. Sautee them until the onion becomes translucent.
3. Rinse the beans, and dice the potatoes. Add everything into the instant pot.
4. Then add vegetable broth and diced tomatoes.
5. Add the ground flax seeds.
6. Add the Indian seasoning blend.
7. Adjust your pressure cooker to high pressure, seal and cook for around 30min.

46. Chicken Pot Pie Soup

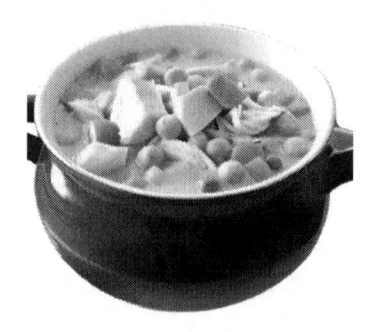

Total: 40 mins

Servings: 4

Ingredients

- 4 boneless, skinless chicken breasts
- 2 tablespoons butter (or coconut oil for dairy-free option)
- Celtic sea salt and freshly ground black pepper

FOR THE SOUP:

- 3 tablespoons unsalted butter (or 2 tablespoons coconut oil for dairy-free)
- 1 yellow onion, chopped
- 3 carrots, chopped

- 3 stalks celery, chopped
- 4 cloves garlic, minced
- 1/2 teaspoon dried thyme
- 2 tablespoons coconut flour
- 1 tablespoon arrowroot flour
- 4 1/2 cups chicken stock
- 1 teaspoon celtic sea salt
- 1 cup frozen green peas, thawed
- 1/2 cup heavy cream (or coconut milk for dairy-free)
- 1/4 cup chopped fresh, flat-leaf parsley
- Juice of 1 lemon

Directions

1. Heat a large pot over medium, add the butter, and swirl to coat the bottom of the pan. Season the chicken breasts with salt and pepper on each side and then place in the pot.
2. Cook until just turning golden brown on the edges, about 4 minutes. Using a pair of tongs, flip the chicken and continue cooking until cooked

through, about 4 minutes. Transfer the chicken to a clean plate and cover to keep warm.

3. Place the butter in the now empty pot and melt over medium heat. Stir in the onion, carrots and celery, reduce the heat to low, and cover and cook for 30 minutes.

4. Stir in the garlic and thyme and cook until fragrant, about 45 seconds. Sprinkle in coconut flour and arrowroot flour, stirring constantly, until absorbed, about 1 minute. Add 1/2 cup stock and cook, stirring constantly, until mixture is thickened, about 1 minute.

5. Stir in the remaining stock, sea salt, and peas. Increase the heat to high and bring to a low boil. While mixture is coming to a boil, shred the chicken and then add to the soup, along with any juices that have accumulated on the plate. Reduce heat to low and stir in cream, parsley and lemon juice. Season with salt to taste.

47. Lemon Chicken and Vegetable Soup

Total: 1 hr 10 mins

Servings: 4

Ingredients

- 4 tablespoons unsalted butter or 3 tablespoons ghee or coconut oil for dairy-free
- 4 carrots, cut into coins
- 4 celery stalks, cut into bite-size pieces
- 1 onion, chopped
- 2 zucchini, cut into 1" thick pieces
- 4 cloves garlic, sliced
- 3 boneless, skinless chicken breasts
- 6 cups bone broth or meat stock
- 1 1/2 tbs grey Celtic sea salt
- 1/4 tsp freshly ground black pepper
- 4 large egg yolks
- 3 tablespoons fresh lemon juice
- 1/2 cup parsley, chopped

Directions

1. Place the butter in a large pot over low heat and melt. Add the carrots, celery, onion, zucchini and garlic to the pot. Stir and then put the lid on the pot and let sweat for 30 minutes.
2. Add the chicken breasts, broth, salt and pepper and bring to a boil over high heat. Reduce heat to medium-low and continue to simmer until chicken is cooked through, about 8 minutes. Using a pair of tongs, remove the chicken and place on a cutting board. Cut the chicken into bite-size pieces and then add back to the broth mixture.
3. In a small bowl, whisk together the egg yolks and lemon juice. Slowly add 1/2 cup of the hot liquid to the egg yolks while whisking constantly. Then, slowly add the yolk mixture to the soup while whisking constantly.
4. Add the parsley, season with additional sea salt and pepper if needed, and serve.

48. Butternut Squash Soup

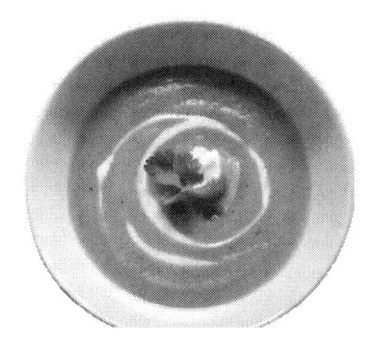

Total: 1 hr

Servings: 4 – 6

Ingredients

- 4 tablespoons ghee, divided
- 4 shallots, chopped
- 1 large butternut squash, peeled and cut into large bite-size pieces
- 1/2 teaspoon Celtic sea salt plus more for seasoning
- 1 teaspoon dried thyme
- 6 cups chicken stock (homemade preferred)
- 1/2 cup coconut milk

Directions

1. Preheat oven to 400°F and adjust rack to middle position. Place 2 tablespoons ghee in a large pot over medium heat. Add shallots and stir. Reduce heat to low, cover pot with a lid and cook for 20 minutes.
2. Toss butternut squash with remaining 2 tablespoons melted ghee and spread evenly on a large baking dish. Season with sea salt. Roast for 15 minutes. Using a spatula, flip the butternut pieces and then roast for an additional 15 minutes, or until the squash is golden brown on the outside and soft on the inside.
3. Stir dried thyme into shallot mixture until fragrant, about 30 seconds. Pour in stock and add butternut squash. Bring to a simmer and cook for 15 minutes. Using a hand-immersion blender, blend soup until smooth (or you can spoon the soup into a blender and blend until smooth). Stir in coconut milk and season with sea salt. Serve.

49. White Bean Soup with Ham
Total: 6 hrs

Servings: 3

Ingredients

FOR THE BEANS:

- 1 pound dried white navy beans
- Pinch of baking soda

FOR THE SOUP:

- 2 meaty smoked ham hocks (pastured preferred)
- 8 cups chicken stock
- 6 ribs celery, cut into bite-size pieces
- 6 carrots, cut into 1/2"-thick coins
- 1 yellow onion, chopped
- 10 cloves garlic, peeled and smashed
- 6 sprigs fresh thyme
- 2 teaspoons Celtic sea salt

Directions

1. The night before, place the white beans in a large bowl and cover with water. Stir in a pinch of baking soda.
2. The next day, drain and rinse the beans and then place them in a slow cooker. Add the ham hocks, chicken stock, celery, carrots, onion, garlic, and thyme in the slow cooker and stir to combine. Cover and cook for about 6 hours on low until the beans are tender.
3. Using a pair of tongs, remove the thyme and ham hocks. Shred the ham and return it back to the slow cooker. Stir in the salt, taste and add more if needed. Serve.

50. Beef Stew

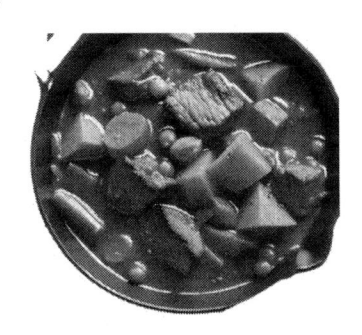

Total: 1 hr

Servings: 6

Ingredients

- 2 tablespoons ghee, divided
- 4 yellow onions, sliced thin
- 2 tablespoons coconut flour
- 2 cloves garlic, minced
- 1 teaspoon dried thyme
- 1 1/2 cups dry white wine (you can substitute this with chicken stock)
- 1 1/2 cups chicken stock
- 3 pounds beef chuck, trimmed and cut into 1 1/2-inch pieces

- 1 tablespoon honey
- 1 tablespoon cider vinegar
- 2 bay leaves
- 2 teaspoons Celtic sea salt
- 1 tablespoon Dijon mustard
- 1/4 cup chopped flat-leaf parsley

Directions

1. Preheat the oven to 250°F and place rack on middle-low position. Heat 2 tablespoons ghee in a large dutch oven (an ovenproof pot with a lid) over medium-low heat.
2. Add the add onions and sauté, stirring frequently until onions release their liquid, about 10 minutes. (If the bottom of the pot begins to brown too much, push the onions aside with a spoon, pour a small amount of water and scrape up the brown bits.)
3. Continue to cook until the onions caramelize, about 15 minutes. Stir in coconut flour and cook for 1 minute. Make a well in the center of the pot

and add garlic and thyme and cook until fragrant, about 45 seconds. Add the wine and chicken stock, scraping up any brown bits on the bottom of the pan. Add the beef, honey, cider vinegar, bay leaves and sea salt. Bring to a boil, cover with the lid and place in the oven. Cook for 2 1/2 hours, until meat is tender. Stir in mustard and parsley and additional sea salt to taste. Serve alone or over creamy mashed potatoes.

Printed in Great Britain
by Amazon